DISCLAIMER

The characters in these stories are purely imaginary and of the author's own imagination. Any resemblance to any characters either living or dead is purely coincidental. Nothing in the content should be used as a substitute for professional medical advice. I can only guide you and create awareness, because any doctor cannot give proper diagnosis and treatment, unless and until they see the patient. You should always visit your general physician for diagnosis and treatment for your specific medical needs.

I would like to dedicate this book to my parents, who are responsible for encouraging me to take up medical course. And also my wife, who supported me a lot for this article.

I would like to convey my special thanks to,

Mr. Rahul, Mr.Sathish, Mr.M.Sounthar

Mr. and Mrs. Dheepakh

Mrs. Hemamalini

Mrs. Rohini Baskaran Deepan

Family Health and well Being – Volume 1

Author – Dr. V. M. Anantha Eashwar

Copyright ©2015 Eashwaranand

FAMILY HEALTH AND WELL BEING : Volume -1

Table of Contents

ALCOHOLISM AND ROAD TRAFFIC ACCIDENTS 4

FEVER 24

SMOKING AND ITS ILL EFFECTS ON VARIOUS SYSTEMS IN OUR BODY 37

ALCOHOLISM AND ROAD TRAFFIC ACCIDENTS

This story tells the story of a John – a chronic alcoholic, and a parallel story of a family of three from a lower socioeconomic status. Both the stories are told in separate sequences and how they meet and the outcome of it in the final sequence. It tells about the outcome of road traffic accidents and head injuries. It tells about how money, power and greed could destroy not only your life, but also others.

SEQUENCE 1

So John, 21 years old was studying his college when he had feelings for a girl Emily in his college. She was his junior in the college and they met during the college function days. On Valentine's Day, he proposed to her. She was initially skeptical whether to accept, but deep inside, she too was having feelings for him. John was tall and was the macho man in the class. He was born into a rich family. His parents were abroad and he was being taken care by his aunt since 4 years old. They would come over to meet him thrice in a year.

Emily was like a girl next door. She was the only child to her parents, who were physicians. Her father – Dr. Raghav, was a former boxing champion and a psychiatrist by profession. Her mother, Sandhya was a general physician.

Any guy would fall for Emilia, the moment they set their eyes along her. But she was a reserved type who doesn't speak much with the boys. As said above John and Emily met during the party days in their school days. Practically, they knew nothing about each other. The only thing they knew about each other were that John was a macho man in the school and Emily was a girl next door.

As John was under the care of his aunt, he didn't receive a mother's warmth or his dad's love. His aunt barely spent time with him. He always spent time with his friends, going to parties, hanging out with the girls. He started consuming alcohol from the age of 19. He also smokes cigarettes frequently. On the other hand, Emily had been just the opposite. She liked her parents a lot and was spending time with them most of the time. She occasionally went to parties…

So on Valentine 'day, Emily was called by a mutual friend to both John and Emily, for her birthday party. They arrived and after the party on a rainy night, John thought it would be the perfect time to propose to her. He proposed to her. She was shocked. She never expected a proposal from one of the most handsome and macho men in the class. She accepted it.

So days passed by. They grew close to each other. John was the dominating type. He wanted Emily to listen to what he says and he never asked her what she wanted. Emily was the adjusting type. She went where and all John wanted her to come with, to movies, to parties and all. He never asked Emily where she would like to go.

John wanted to go with Emily for a long drive on the highway. Emily didn't like the idea as she was afraid of travelling by bike on highway and knowing that John had a racing bike, it feared her more. And that's what thrilled John more and more, to see her screaming when he travelled at high speed. It was going to be an adventure for him. So they planned to go by the weekend. Emily had to tell lies in her home, to go out. John had consumed alcohol on the night before at a party.

The day arrived, John woke up in the morning and he was feeling a little dizzy. But he ignored it and started from his home to pick up Emily. Emily was waiting near her college gate. When she came to know that he was a little sleepy, she refused to go with him. She told him to take some rest and that they can reschedule for a later date. He didn't even have helmets on him. John said that he had been waiting this day for so long. He acted as if he was crying. Emily couldn't stand to see him in tears. So she accepted and they started on his long awaited journey. John was initially driving at slow speeds at 70kmph and was starting to feel a little dizzy.

Emily was talking to him about her family, her dream post marriage and all. John asked Emily that if she would want an unforgettable thrilling experience. Emily understood what he meant and begged him not to go at high speeds. But John, in spite of her warnings started to speed his bike. Since it was a racing bike he was going at 100,110,140,170 and finally he was travelling at 180kmph. Emily was shouting in fear, to slow down the bike. John saw someone in scooter driving at a slow speed. He purposefully increased his speed to show off and reached 200kmph and passed by a motor scooter.

SEQUENCE 2

There was a family of three, a married couple - Ram, Nithya, and their son Suresh. Suresh was 7 years old. Ram and Nithya were 40 and 39 years respectively. Nithya didn't conceive till 8 years after marriage. She conceived through intrauterine fertilization (IUI) after 8 years of marriage. They were both very much caring for their son. Suresh was studying in his school. They wanted their son to study in the best of the best schools. So they got a loan and spent all their savings to put him in one of the top rated schools in the city. Ram worked day and night to earn money. Nithya was a caring housewife who took care of Suresh and Ram. Everyone envied for the happiness and positive energy in their family.

Both of them (Ram and Nithya) had a good understanding of each other. Suresh was the topper in his class, and also the teachers used to like him very much due to his obedience, punctuality, and regularity. Suresh loves his parents a lot. Whatever the day is whatever the situation is how much ever tired he is, he needs his mother beside him to get a good day's sleep. They didn't have any vehicle. How much ever the travelling distance is, they used to walk or travel by buses. Ram gathered money, day by day to buy at least a motor scooter, so that he could drop his son in his school. So one day when Suresh was 12 years old, Ram came home with a newly bought scooter. Everyone was so happy. Ram used to take Suresh in his scooter every day, to drop him in school.

One day they plan to go to a theme park on a weekend. They went to a bus terminus and saw that all the buses were full. Suresh was disappointed. But he didn't tell anything to his parents. They reached home. Suresh took a book from his bag and started to study. His mother could understand Suresh's disappointment. When he was reading his book, a tear from his eye fell on the book. He immediately wiped them and said to his parents that something had fell in his eye and he started to wipe them away.

Her mother couldn't see his son in tears. She immediately went to Ram and asked him whether he could do anything. Ram, even called all the taxis to check their availability and none of them were available. Then Ram stood up. He told Suresh to get ready as they are leaving by scooter. Nithya asked whether it would be safe to travel with three in a scooter, but Ram replied that he would be travelling only at low speed only and asked her not to worry. Suresh was very happy. Everyone got ready and they were ready to leave. Ram started the scooter and with Suresh in the middle with Ram and Nithya on the front and back respectively, they started their journey. They reached the highways. Ram was driving in the sides, and he was merely driving at the rate of 50kmph for his family's safety. Behind him, he heard a roaring side of a bike with a girl shouting.

FINAL SEQUENCE

As John wanted to scare the scooter guy, he drove up in high speed. But John lost control of his bike. He immediately tried to lower his speed and lowered up to 100kmph, which caused his bike to skid. John's elbow hit on the ground with a crackling sound. Emily's arm and head rubbed against the road. After the bike hit the scooter drove by Ram, Emily fell on the ground and rotating hand bar and the tires of the bike hit her in the face and threw her away. The impact threw the scooter away; the impact threw Ram over a roadblock with his back against it. He immediately fell unconscious. Nithya knows that the accident was inevitable, she hugged her son and the impact threw her to the ground and she was going a few meters on the road before her head hit the roadblock. As she was hugging her son, he was shielded from the impact except his head which hit on the ground. Emily's face was covered in blood with some of her hair torn from the scalp. Nithya had abrasions all over the side of the body against which she fell on the road. She was dizzy. She called her son and asked whether he was okay and asked him to check on Ram. Ram was unconscious and after repeated shouting by Suresh, Ram opened his eyes partially, but was unable to move. Suresh started to cry and he ran to his mother who was struggling to even move. He held her hands and begged her to wake up. She immediately held her hand over her head and shouted in pain after which she became unconscious holding his hand. And finally John had his hand and legs trapped under the bike and was shouting for help and was shouting Emily's name and crying. There was no reply from Emily, other than a faint movement in her hands and foot.

Persons nearby called the ambulance as soon as they saw the incident and emergency vehicles came and picked everyone up and transported them to a nearby multi-specialty hospital.

Suresh couldn't stop his tears. Just before a few minutes, everyone was happily chatting, in just half an hour, his world turned upside down. All the five of them, including Suresh were sent to take an MRI scan of the brain. But Suresh refused as he had only a minor abrasion in the hands and legs. He begged the doctors to do the scan, first for his parents and let him know the results. Preliminary tests began and the scan was done for them. They were all sent to an intensive care unit in a semiconscious state and the doctors continued with the procedure for them.

Emily's parents were working there, so as soon as they heard the condition of Emily they rushed to the ICU to check the progress of their child. The doctors came out of the ICU. They apologized to Suresh that they could not save his parents. They told Suresh that his parents have suffered head injuries and as a result, they passed away a few minutes ago. Suresh was in absolute silence. He was sitting near Emily's mother- Dr.Radha. She thought that he was going to break in tears. But he stood up and started walking. Emily's father – Dr.

Raghav told his wife to check on him and he said that he will take care of Emily. Radha immediately stood up and was running towards Suresh. Suresh was feeling dizzy and he stood near a staircase and was calling his Mom and Dad to take him with them and was about to fall down. Radha rushed to him and caught him. She asked the doctors whether the MRI scan was performed and they replied that he did not have any symptoms pertaining to head injury. Radha shouted at the doctors to perform MRI scan immediately. Then, she came back to check on Emily. Chief Doctor came and narrated the incidents which would have happened leading to this accident. They asked how Emily was progressing. The doctors told that Emily developed an intracranial hemorrhage and she has only a few minutes before she could pass out. Radha couldn't control her tears. The radiologist came and told Radha that Suresh passed away during the scan procedure as he was bleeding inside his brain due to the impact. Though Nithya tried her best to protect him, a single impact to the head at such a high speed is enough to cause bleeding inside the brain.

Raghav went inside the ICU and sat down near Emily and held her hands. He said to her, "Baby doll, I don't know whether you could hear me. But remember, your mom and I had always loved you and we always will. You are going to a safe place. Don't forget about us. You always wanted to save people and that's why you took this profession. It's not your mistake for this accident. Accidents happen. Due to your kind nature God has called you soon." Suddenly Emily held his hands and tapped his palm with her fingers. She began moaning and suddenly she started spitting blood and her ECG turned Flat line. Raghav knew that her soul passed away. The only child, he had, his source of happiness, his dreams of seeing her married, hugging his grandchildren, all turned to ashes in just a 3 second time. He could hear his wife crying outside. He slowly left her hands and could see her soulless body lying on the bed. He didn't drop a single tear. He didn't speak anything.

He went to his home with his wife after finishing all the formalities. He came and sat on the sofa and stared at the ceiling. Radha continued crying. She went to Emily's room and hugged all her belongings. Raghav closed his eyes. All he could think of was Emily. The day, which she walked, the day she first called his dad, the days she cared for him during the boxing matches, the day they had good times. He opened his eyes. He burst out in tears and shouted EMILY! Radha on hearing that ran to him and hugged him. Two days passed. He went to the hospital.

He directly went to John's room. He saw him lying in the bed and inquired the doctors about his condition. They replied that he had fractured one of his leg and hand and had multiple abrasions over his face. They said it would take at least 1 year for his full recovery including rehabilitation. Raghav asked whether he could have a few words with him and went to John. He was lying in the bed, staring at the ceiling. John was with his parents who came to visit him from abroad on hearing the incident. John's father - Brad was one of the top businessmen. Brad came and apologized to Raghav. He didn't reply to anything. Raghav sat near John and asked him why he took Emily out that day, for which he replied, "Sir, I love Emily with all my heart. She is everything to me. I wanted to live with her till my last breath. I never expected this to happen. Please forgive me, Sir." Raghav replied "That's all I wanted to know" and he left.

So years passed by. Radha went into depression. One day Raghav wakes up in the morning and got ready to go to the hospital. Radha didn't wake up yet. He went to check on her and found her body as cold as ice. He immediately called the emergency crew and checked for a pulse and found none. He went and took the stethoscope from his room, checked for her heartbeat and found none. The emergency crew arrived and she was rushed to the hospital. As a doctor Raghav knew the result. He lay down in his bed. After a few minutes, he received a call from the hospital that her wife passed away due to cardiac arrest.

He took his car, went to the hospital. She was in the intensive care unit, just like his daughter was, three years ago. He could see the soulless body lying on the bed. The only person whom he cared about and the only person who cared about him passed away. He went to his quarters in the hospital and fainted.

He woke up in the hospital bed. The hospital staff immediately called the chief doctor about seeing his wake. The chief came and checked his condition and told "Your loss is unbearable. How many patients you would have treated for depression? How many families you would have saved doctor? God has a purpose for each and every human being. You will find that soon. Stay in your hospital quarters till you feel well. If you have any problems, I am all ears. I am a surgeon. How many lives I would have saved? The person who are undergoing the surgery, with a maximum of ten persons per day. How many lives you are saving each and every day? You save at least ten families with your psychotherapy. Think of what are all the things you told to people who were victims of depression." And the chief left the room.

Years passed by. It was the day of Emily's graduation, if she would have been alive. He waited for this day, since the day she joined her college. He waited for the day she would enter the house and hug him and tell that she became a doctor. Now he sat on the chair, staring at the entrance of his house. The next day morning, at around 7 AM he went for a walk. He received a call from the hospital that he had many appointments in the morning. He told that he would be coming by 10 AM. He was about to enter a hotel to have the breakfast, when he saw four bikes speeding behind him. All the four bike riders were wearing helmets with each of them having a girl behind. John followed them into a hotel. He covered his face partially with his cap and sat near their table. All of them were talking about some trekking and all.

To his surprise, he identifies one of them as John, the same person who ran into an accident with his daughter which led to the demise of his daughter and a family of 3. He closely watched his activities. The girl who sat behind him on his bike was standing near John. John stood up. He removed his cap, so that to check whether John identifies him. Everyone turned towards Raghav.

John said "Oh, Doctor. How are you? You are that girl's father right? What is her name? Something like Emi- Emilia right? Your girl was one of the best I ever dated, what a girl she was! Sadly, she had to die that day. She literally begged me not to go for the ride that day. But I didn't listen, my bad. What is it? You are not angry at me? You are standing like a zombie! I heard about your wife Sorry for your loss. I can't understand. Why is she so important to you people? She died in an accident. Get over it! Enjoy your life" Raghav had no words to speak. Raghav clenched his fists and knocked him out with a single punch.

John woke up. He was feeling dizzy and had a headache. He found himself sitting on a chair with his hands tied to the back. It was dark. He shouted Raghav's name. He threatened Raghav, that he will tell his parents and he would be behind bars in no time. The lights came back on, he found himself in a room familiar from his past. It was a girl's room. It had John's photos all over the place. Then he remembered that it was Emilia's room. He had heard her tell him how she decorated her room. He looked around and found Raghav standing in one corner.

Raghav comes over and sits in a chair in front of John. Raghav tells, "How are you John? It's been nearly 5 years. How was your life all these years? Dating, hanging out with friends, drinking, smoking, and everything right." John speaks "Hey doctor, that's how a person of my age and my status should be! So you are going to kill me right? Like in movies! The father of the girl comes and tortures and kills the person responsible and gives a wicked laugh and he himself will commit suicide when the police arrive. Am I right?"

"Now listen to me John. This will get over soon if you just shut up and sit for as long as I say. So what are the things you remember of the incident that day, which killed my child and a family of three?"

John replied "See, doctor. I was drunk. I was feeling dizzy. I was driving at high speed and I lost my control which led to that accident. I never wanted Emily to die that day. I just wanted to show off. It was an accident. That family, I don't know who they were. I don't care. I asked my father to take care of them. And for Emily, I never ever loved her. That day when you came to visit me, I told like that because my parents were there beside me that day. In fact, I never loved any girl in my life, and none of the girls ever loved me for my character or anything. They all acted as if they loved me only for my physical looks and my money. There is nothing called true love. After some years pass, I will marry a girl as per my likes and live with her. I have power, I have money and I can buy anything in this world. So if you could please untie me, I will act as if this never happened and be on my way. Am I clear doctor?"

Raghav replied "So this is what you had to say. Okay. So I will tell a small background of your family. Your parents live abroad. You were brought up by your aunt. You don't know about the values of friendship, family, and money. You try to show off and buy people with your money and that is why you don't have any real friends. You think all are with you only for your money. Since you do favors for your friends, you expect them to obey you and do whatever you tell them to. They don't care for you. I will now show a sample. So tell me any of your friends whom you think will do anything for you."

John replied "Whatever you told in the beginning may be correct. Who told you that I don't have real friends? Take my mobile and call any of my friends and see. You don't know anything about friendship. You want to know about my friends? Call and see. I won't interfere." Raghav took John's mobile and called one of his friends and put him on loudspeaker, "Is it Karthik? I found someone named John lying on the street unconscious. I knew his name by his ID card. Your number was on his mobile in his recent call history. Do you know him? He is not breathing. I think he may be dead. I was not able to reach the emergency helpline. Can you come over to my place and take him to the hospital?" The voice replied, "Hey old man I don't know what you are talking about. Now get lost" and he disconnected

John was shocked. He had no words to express. Raghav spoke, "This is what you call friendship? You cannot buy friendship. You have to earn it. And your money and status Have you ever earned a single penny in your life? You have lived only on your parent's money and the luxuries they gave you. I don't want to break this to you, but if I would have called your parents and told the same, their reaction may be similar to what your friend said. So you don't have a family and you don't have friends. You lack the two most important part of each and every human life. And what if you marry a girl? You would be having kids. What if they die in the same way Emily died? What will you do then? Or else you want to raise them up in the same way as you were raised. This world is so huge. If I ask you to tell even one person in this world who cares about you, you can't. So why do you need to live? With all this money you have, have you spent them on doing any good deeds? No! Entertainment and Enjoyment were your two important aspects of your life. If you die, there must be at least a single living soul, who could shed a tear for you. If not, the reason for your existence in this world is totally meaningless. So now we have agreed that you don't have either a family who care for you or real friends. Each and every one you know is going to ditch you. And relationships! What do you know about them?

So you didn't love Emily right? Have a look around her room. She had photos of you. She loved you with all her heart. She always had the habit of writing her diary. I will read some pages from her diary. "I met him for the first time in my college. He seemed lost. Though he is happy and all, his eyes showed sadness. I want to know more about him."

A few pages later "He proposed to me. I didn't know what to say. I accepted. Not because of his money and looks. He is just the opposite of my character. He has a lot of bad habits. He is a chronic alcoholic and a smoker. The reason he is like, this is because of his parents. Whatever important work they would have had, his mother should have been with him. He is a spoilt child. I have belief that I can change him with my care and affection. I will give him the love and care his parents never gave him. He is my first love. I don't want his money or anything. Even if we live in a small home, I can make it happy. Whatever fights we have, whatever misunderstandings we have, I will never leave him. I have to speak with my father about this. Tomorrow he has called me for a drive on the highway. I am afraid of it. But he is stubborn. I will not disappoint him. Hope he understands my feelings soon. Right now we have to concentrate on our studies. I want him to become a psychiatrist like my father. That's when he will meet all kinds of people. That's when he will understand what life is. Whatever fights we have in our family, he takes only 2 minutes to settle things down. My daddy is my hero. I have to sleep early.

Tomorrow is a big day for me. I am going to tell all my feelings to him. I hope I am ready for it."

He read the diary and kept it aside and saw John. He went and untied him. John didn't try to escape. He was sitting in his chair, without speaking anything. Raghav continued, "You can't be on your father's shadow always. You have to create an identity for yourself. Life is full of opportunities. Make use of them. Earn respect by giving respect to others. You want to know about the family you hit that day? They had only one son and were from a lower middle class family. Their son was their life and soul. They lived to make him happy, they worked hard to make him happy. Their life ended in just 5 seconds. His mother suffered severe spinal cord injuries as she was trying to protect her son while falling. She also suffered a severe brain hematoma. His father's spinal cord broke in half. And the son was conscious till he came to know that his parents were dead. After his parent's died, he begged each and everyone in the hospital that he wants his parents back. He wants to hear their voice again and he can't sleep without his mother. But the concussion he had suffered during the fall led to internal bleeding in his brain, which led to his demise. The last words he spoke were, "Mom, its paining a lot, please help me". Think of the things which would have been going through his mind in his last few minutes. Do you know how many people are like you in this city? Each and every week one death or the other happens like this. Families are getting destroyed. Dreams are getting destroyed. But all you people think are the thrills and adventures. The situation has to change. Don't know when that will happen. You can leave, John. Kill as many as you wish. But each and every bad deed you do, you will get punished in this life in one way or the other. Learn to accept your mistakes. At least have some feelings. The only wrong judgment I made in my life is that I thought that you loved Emily. The only wrong thing that Emily did in her life was, to fall for you and thought that she could change you."

John stood up. He asked Raghav whether he could borrow Emily's diary for a day. Raghav handed it to John, who turned and left. He went to his home and started reading her diary. Each and every line he read brought tears to his eyes. Next day morning at around 10 am, he departed from his home to hand over the diary to Raghav. There was heavy traffic near Raghav's house. John got down from his vehicle, and inquired. They said that someone died in a house nearby. John rushed to Raghav's house. When he reached there he found that Raghav has passed away due to cardiac arrest. He saw Raghav's body being taken for funeral. He followed them. He saw nearly thousands of people, gathered for his funeral. Each and every one was his patients. John remembered Raghav's words, "You have to earn respect. If you die there must be at least one person to shed a tear for you." There he saw hundreds of people shedding tears for him. After his funeral he went to his home and called his father and asked for a huge amount of money.

After nearly 20 years, a chronic alcoholic is being taken by his family in a car in a semiconscious state. His whole family is crying. They get down from the car to take him to a place. The sign read:

"Dr. John's de-addiction and rehabilitation center" Once entered there was a huge statue of Dr. Raghav with a note written,

This hospital is dedicated to Dr. Raghav, my inspiration and my role model and my hero.

Today whatever position I am in is because of you and Emily – Dr. John, Psychiatrist and social activist.

FEVER

Fever is a very broad term. So what is a fever? As we all know in simple terms, an increase in our body temperature! What do we do to get well of that fever? Normally we don't go to the doctor. We go to the pharmacy and buy some medicines to reduce the fever and we settle with the temporary wellbeing. When the incident occurs more than three or four times, then we only think of going to the doctor.

In my general practice, I have seen only a few patients coming with the complaints of fever for the past duration of within 24 hours. What they don't have is "Awareness".

We always take "fever" lightly. We think that, it will go away if I take medications for reducing the fever and I will get cured. We will get a temporary reduction in fever, that's for sure, sometimes it may not even re-occur, Note the point, "Sometimes" you won't get relief from the fever even after taking over the counter fever reducing medicines, which are readily available in the pharmacy. I am not saying that you have to go to a doctor immediately if you suspect fever. But "the cause of fever" That's what you have to care.

So I am going to tell a small story about "what may happen if you ignore your fever without treating the cause of it!"

So let's start with a family of three. A 6 year old son named John and their parents being Victor and Emily respectively. Victor and Emily got married. And at the age of 22 years they had their son, the year following their marriage.

When John was about 5 years old, he was feeling slightly warm over his forehead; their parents suspected fever and gave him fever reducing medications. John started feeling well and started to play and run around the house, his parents were feeling happy and left as it is. The next day he developed some headache and was again feeling warm. So they gave him the same medication and the fever got reduced and they were doing the same again and again for 3 days. Day by day the time duration between the fever reducing medication and the time he develops a fever got increased.

4th DAY:

On the 4th day he developed shivering, which was followed by sweating and he was too weak to play. Also, he developed a dry cough, which is nothing but **"cough without expectoration"** i.e. cough without spitting sputum and some mild abdominal pain. So his parents noticed that something is wrong with him and took him to a doctor. The doctor checked him and asked the symptoms and the duration of fever and whether he has abdominal pain, difficulty in passing urine, any loose stools or dysentery (Blood in stools) and he was prescribed with fever reducing medication along with antibiotics and asked if they would want to do some blood investigations for diagnosing the type of fever. They replied "no" as he had fever only for duration of 4 days, the parents said.

The Antibiotics are the drugs which fight against the organisms which are responsible for causing the infection, which means only the bacteria and not against the virus, fungi and parasites. So the doctor prescribed the medicines for 3 days and asked them to come to his clinic the next day to check the progress of the illness. But they ignored the next two days and did not take him to the doctor.

6th DAY:

The next two days John was feeling somewhat better, but he was still too weak to play and he had mild stomach pain. This puts the parents in worry, and they took him to the same doctor. Note that it is the 6th day of his illness. So the doctor checked and urged them to immediately do some blood investigations, to check what type of fever he was having. So he wrote some blood tests which I will explain in detail.

The parents were skeptical, whether to do all these tests as the cost is high. But they accept it and did these tests and they were requested to come and collect the results on the following day. **Hb, TC, DC, ESR, Platelet count, Urine routine examination, MP by QBC.** So what are these tests?

Hb – Hemoglobin – to check the amount of hemoglobin, the child had. Low hemoglobin can cause anemia, which in turn can cause weakness, headache.

TC – It is **total count** of the white blood cells, which are the "police force of our body" They are increased in case of bacterial infection and decreased in case of viral infections.

DC – Differential white blood cell count, which shows the amount of neutrophils, Basophils, Lymphocytes and Easinophils, which are the components of white blood cells and any variation in one of them can give an idea of what infection it might be.

ESR – *Erythrocyte Sedimentation Rate* This will be increased in all types of active bacterial infections.

Urine Routine examination – This will check for any presence of pus cells, which points the diagnosis towards UTI which is urinary tract infections and the presence of blood in urine, which may point to any presence of infection in kidney or UTI or any urinary bladder infections.

MP by QBC – These tests are for the presence of malarial parasites in blood.

Platelet count – It is an important component. It helps in the clotting of blood. Any decrease in the platelet count accompanied by body pain and fever, dengue fever must be suspected. Any abnormal decrease of which can point to a diagnosis like dengue, which left untreated, can lead to life threatening complications.

Widal - It is a blood test to diagnose typhoid fever caused by an organism called Salmonella Typhi.

7th DAY:

The next morning his parents woke up and were searching for John, who usually will be playing around. But what they saw was shocking. They saw their son was standing in front of a mirror and speaking to his reflection. Victor asked John, who you are speaking to. John replied that he is speaking to his grandfather and playing with him in the park! His father gets shocked in horror! At that time, Victor's father was passed away 2 years ago!

Victor gets terrified and lifted John and he called his wife and told her that their son is haunted by a GHOST and they have to take him to a person who specializes in this field. They started the vehicle and went to all the persons whom they know and perform all the rituals to extract the ghost from his body. They are least bothered about the results of the blood tests. And his condition was getting worse minute by minute.

And finally, FINALLY! In the evening they decided to go to the doctor. But they got stuck in traffic. By the time they reach his clinic, it was nearly 10 PM and the doctor has already left. Their son started showing "Altered state of consciousness". His parents put him in their vehicle and rushed to a 24 hours multi-specialty hospital and as soon as they reached hospital their son started throwing seizures (fits). Victor carried his son in his arms and with tears in his eyes, he screamed for the doctor, who immediately administered emergency medications to control the seizures and transferred John to an Intensive care unit. The doctor came and asked the history in detail, including the haunting incidents, which happened in the morning. The doctor asked his parents not to worry, and they were performing the blood investigations to find out the type of fever.

8th DAY:

Early in the morning, the doctor came in and told their parents to relax. The blood reports have come, they diagnosed what type of fever and they were doing the necessary treatment to John.

The parents asked the doctor what type of fever it was. The doctor replied that it was MALARIA. Victor shouted in anger, do you think I am a fool? Do I look like a Stupid for you? I recently had malaria and had treatment for it and it was nothing like which my son is having right now". The doctor replied "Calm down Victor, your son is not having any ordinary type of malaria; he is having a dangerous, fatal type of malaria known as **"CEREBRAL MALARIA"**

    Victor apologized to the doctor and asked what that was? And the doctor explained everything and said that you should thank god that your son didn't go into coma. As it would have complicated things and it would have caused irreversible brain damage.

John gets better in a week's time and goes home feeling better. Also the story ends.

Wait, why did I tell this story to you?

I will explain all the details from the beginning of this story and what **should have been done** and what **should have not been done**

So what are these tests?

Now I would like to tell some facts from a doctor's point of view of this story.

So let us take the events happening in the story from the beginning,

John had a fever for 3 days and didn't go to the doctor.

Having a fever for 3 days and not taking treatment, is that OK! If it is okay, what's the reason for it?

Because, our body has an immune system, correct? To fight off infections, correct? So in order for it to work properly, we need to let it do its thing. How?

Let me give you an example "A kid is learning to ride a bicycle; he will fall down every time in the beginning. Finally, he will ride it like everybody" Our immune system is like that only. It has to learn to fight infections.

4th day of fever

So on the 4th day of fever, he developed shivering, which was followed by sweating, which is a typical characteristic feature of malarial fever. So first, what is shivering? In case of malaria fever, shivering typically means teeth chattering and the person will be covered in sheets. During cold seasons we will be covered in sheets that are completely different from shivering in case of malarial fever. So in what other conditions that shivering manifest? Urinary tract infections, any abscess (pus filled boils anywhere in the body when left untreated) anywhere in the body and in a typical malarial fever.

So he had a dry cough, which is nothing to worry about, as it would be due to many infections or it would have been even allergic cough.

He had some mild abdominal pain, that's ok you may think as having fever will cause stomach upset and all but abdominal pain is a very broad term and it may also take the diagnosis in completely different path. But the child's complaint is abdominal pain, the question arises, where is the abdominal pain?

- If the abdominal pain is in the epigastrium (center in the midline of the chest just where the stomach starts), it may take the diagnosis towards gastritis, which is not typically considered in a 6 year old child.

- If there is lower abdominal pain, it may point the diagnosis towards urinary tract infections.

- If there is pain in the left and right side of the stomach while passing stools, it may point the diagnosis towards Amoebiasis (which is an infection caused by an amoeba and it will surely be followed by diarrhea or in some cases there will be even blood in stools).
- Abdominal pain on the right side may indicate problems in the liver.

- Abdominal pain in left side may indicate problems in the spleen or gall bladder.

So if I start to explain all the causes of abdominal pain, then there will be no end to this article. So let's see this case.

Fever + Shivering followed by sweating + Abdominal pain on left side - may point the diagnosis towards malarial fever, but we have to confirm it by blood investigations.

So the parents refused to do the blood test, that's okay for any parent refusing to see their son to get pricked for a blood test. So the doctor prescribed some medicines and asked them to come next day. That's what most doctors do.

6th day of fever.

So on 6th day all blood tests were done and they were asked to collect the results the other day.

First, let me tell you a peculiar thing about the blood test for malaria.

On the day the test being done the parasites should be strong enough and the numbers should be large enough for the test to be positive. So a person having a negative malaria test has a 1 percent chance that the test could be false negative.

Malaria is transmitted by a female Anopheles mosquito and it carries the pathogenic parasite in its salivary glands, so the disease is transmitted to the humans when the mosquito bites the humans. The main pathogenic (means disease causing) parasites causing the disease in humans are Plasmodium vivax and Plasmodium falciparum. Plasmodium is vivax being the common cause of uncomplicated malaria and Plasmodium falciparum being the main culprit, which when left untreated can cause even death.

So most of the time we have a false assumption that malarial fever will not be fatal. The malarial blood test will show which parasite is present in the blood. So any fever which lasts for more than 3 days with shivering, headache, body pain should be suspected for malaria and necessary blood tests should be done for the same.

I am not going to go into the details of the life cycle of malarial parasite as it would be boring. So to be short and precise, Plasmodium falciparum has a characteristic feature of sequestrating the red blood cells and reaching the small blood vessels in the brain, which is responsible for causing the seizures, altered consciousness and in some cases even coma and death. Now let's go to the 7th day.

7th day of fever

So on the seventh day he developed some symptoms which made the parents think that a ghost has haunted him. These symptoms occur when the disease or a pathogen has infiltrated the cells in the brain or it may even be due to conditions like hypoglycemia (low blood sugar level, meningitis (inflammations of the coverings of the brain due to infection). So the parents thought that something was wrong with him and thought he was haunted and took him to people who were specializing in that field and they delayed the treatment till night. That time frame is very important. He could have got seizures any point of time, which would have been followed by coma, so they went to the hospital and got treated in the night.

So I am going to put up some **frequently asked questions** which run in every parent's mind when their son gets affected by any illness, maybe it's a fever or anything and what they should be doing.

1. Should I take my children to a doctor if I suspect fever? - That depends on what the co-existing symptoms are present, like cough with yellow sputum coming from nose or mouth and we have to note the breathing pattern of the child whether it is rapid breathing or not, if the child passes blood in stools , if the child cries while passing urine or if the urine output has decreased compared to before or passes dark colored urine in spite of drinking lot of water, is shivering a lot, if the child has severe headache, when you can hear a whistling sound when the child breathes while sleeping. These are some of the conditions which require a visit to a nearby physician in spite of the

day of fever. And if the child has a history of having seizures when getting high fever at any time during the childhood, known as febrile seizures, then the visit to the physician is mandatory whenever high fever is suspected.

2. Should I be worried about Plasmodium vivax malarial fever, as it says in the report? - All malarial fevers should be treated no matter what the parasite may be involved. In case of Falciparum, no further delay should be made, as treatment should be given as soon as possible.

3. Are all other blood tests really needed? - Yes, all the other blood tests would be equally important to give an idea about what infection it might be.

SMOKING AND ITS ILL EFFECTS ON VARIOUS SYSTEMS IN OUR BODY

So my next topic will be smoking. In general practice, I see a lot of patients who are chronic smokers and some of them are occasional smokers. So what's the difference between these two kinds of people? The difference is nil. In reality, though a chance of developing **COPD** – Chronic Obstructive Pulmonary Disease is high in chronic smokers, the occasional smokers also have the same risk.

"Individual susceptibility" – that's the main factor we have to note. It means that the rate and degree at which smoking affects various systems in our body is different from person to person, which we cannot predict. Each person's body metabolism, lung capacity, chest expansion, genetic expression is different.

So there may be a person who smokes 20 packs a day for 10 years and be healthy without any health issues. There may be another person who smokes only 2 to 3 cigarettes per day for over a period of 10 years and develop COPD or health issues due to that. So there is no use in comparing you to chronic smokers and satisfy you like, "See this person, he smokes 10 packs per day and is healthy. I smoke only 5 cigarettes per day and I am going to be healthy!"

In my general practice, I have seen people telling awesome reasons for smoking like,

- ❖ "Sir, I just stopped taking alcohol sir, this is the only bad habit I have sir, I will stop soon sir", This I think, he has been telling me for nearly 3 years.
- ❖ "Sir, I smoke only in the morning or else I feel constipated sir"
- ❖ "I smoke only when I drink alcohol, sir"
- ❖ "Lots of problems in my home, sir, I smoke to keep my mind at ease sir".
- ❖ And some students, they used to say that they smoke to keep awake at night for late night studies.

These are some of the beliefs people used to have hammered into their brain, that whatsoever you tell them, they won't listen!

Smoking can cause cancer! This is known by many people and they used to think occasional smoking or smoking few cigarettes a day won't harm their body. THEY ARE TERRIBLY WRONG.

Let me tell you a short story to create awareness and to educate people about complications due to smoking.

So there lived a happy couple. Let's name them Victor and Emilia. They were happily married for nearly ten years and lived a healthy married life. Victor was a non-alcoholic, but he was a chronic smoker and he was defending his smoking habit by telling that he smokes to relieve stress. He smokes at work, after every meal and even in the night after his wife sleeps.

They were reaching an age of 35 years and they were planning to have a baby. So they tried to conceive for nearly a year with no luck. Emilia was also suffering from frequent upper respiratory tract infections like cough and sore throat. Then, one fine day, they visited a doctor to address the issue and for consulting. The doctor does the regular infertility tests for both partners. Victor shocked to hear that his blood sugar levels have increased and he has a minor reduction in his sperm count. The doctor spoke to him privately and came to know that he has anxiety issues.

The doctor asked victor for history of smoking and alcohol, and he admits that he smokes a lot of cigarettes per day. The doctor advised him to stop smoking and told him that, it may passively even affect his wife if he smokes when she is around. The doctor prescribed him some drugs for his diabetes. For Emily, all the tests for infertility came back as perfectly normal, except her blood cholesterol levels which were high.

The doctor advised her to reduce fatty diet, to do some exercises and check the cholesterol levels after a month. Victor was hiding the fact to her wife Emilia that, the doctor has advised him to stop smoking.

Days passed on. Victor was searching for possible side effects and the relationship between smoking and low sperm count through the internet, and he finds out. Victor quit smoking for two months. After nearly 3 months Emilia got conceived and she became pregnant. They were so happy and the celebrations began!

Emilia went for regular antenatal checkups and everything was fine until her 7th month. After then her blood pressure started to increase. Doctors started her on prophylactic drugs to avoid hypertension at the time of delivery. During the ultrasound on the 8th month, the amniotic fluid surrounding the child began to decrease (Amniotic fluid supplies the necessary nutrients to the fetus) and goes to a value of 8 (Normal value should be above 9). Doctors advised her to take a lot of oral fluids and monitored her amniotic fluid volume every week. Suddenly, in the 8th month, she was developing labor pains and her blood pressure started to increase. So emergency surgery was done and a baby boy was delivered, but the baby didn't cry after birth. So the baby got admitted in the neonatal care unit and necessary care was given. Victor & Emilia went home with the baby boy after a month of his stay in the neonatal care unit.

They named their baby boy as **John**. Years passed by. John became 5 years old. He was fine, but had a history of Bronchial asthma since birth and was on medication for that. Meanwhile, Victor started to develop high blood pressure at the age of 40. So he was on both Anti-Diabetic and Anti-Hypertensive medications. In spite of doctor's advice to stop smoking, he smokes packs and packs per day.

Once, they went on a holiday picnic with family. After having a heavy meal, Victor noticed some pain in his left arm, radiating to his left shoulder. He took some pain relieving medications and went to sleep. He woke up in the middle of the night gasping for breath and noticed some mild chest pain. He woke his wife. Then she called the ambulance and they immediately rushed him to a hospital. The doctors took an **ECG** and found out that he had a massive heart attack. They admitted him in **ICU** and did the necessary treatment. He was discharged from hospital and the doctor warned him not to smoke again. So let's stop here.

Let me tell you the actual events from the beginning of this story from a doctor's point of view in simple language.

Victor was a chronic smoker. What does a cigarette contain?

It contains nicotine, which is a brain stimulant. When the person inhales smoke, it immediately reaches the lungs and gets absorbed into bloodstream. The nicotine cross the blood-brain barrier and exhibit their **CNS stimulant** (brain stimulant) properties, so the person feels a sense of "high" when smoking.

- Smokers used to say that they smoke to relieve their stress. But in reality, they feel more anxious and irritable during the time interval between smokings. So anxiety disorders are common among smokers, when compared with non- smokers. This may have been the cause of anxiety issues in Victor.

- Smoking can cause erectile dysfunction due to restriction of the blood flow due to thickening of blood vessels. It also exhibits oxidative stress on the sperms which can in turn reduce the sperm count as free radicals could destroy the sperm. This could be the cause of Victor's low sperm count in the beginning.

- Then coming to the most important point – **PASSIVE SMOKING**. Emily may be a non-smoker, but Victor used to smoke in the night after his wife sleeps and even at home. So these harmful gases when inhaled by Emily contribute to Passive smoking. They lived 10 years together, after which she conceived. So she passively smoked for 10 years!

- Smoking in women can lead to premature delivery (Delivery of the fetus before 37 weeks), stillbirth and abortion. So this passive smoking may have even lead to Emily going into premature labor. Smoking in women can even lead to chances of getting cervical cancer and early menopause. So the low birth weight and premature birth of John may have been due to passive smoking by Emily, when Victor smokes at home.

- Smoking cause's high cholesterol and due to the restriction of blood flow can cause a stroke (due to decreased blood supply to the brain), Myocardial infarction (**Heart attack** – maybe due to the restriction of blood flow or high cholesterol causing blockages in the blood vessels). So the reasons for Victor getting a massive heart attack may be attributed to Smoking.

- Passive smoking by John may have led to his condition of frequent upper respiratory tract infections and asthma.

- Victor's symptoms like pain in the left arm, chest pain with sweating and breathlessness are signs of a heart attack.

So smoking may not only cause lung cancer, it may cause damage to all the organ systems in our body.

So comparing yourself to other chronic smokers who are healthy is completely pointless. All the health issues which I mentioned MAY be caused by smoking. I am not saying all smokers will suffer the same health issues; they may or may not get them, as it all depends on their body metabolism, genetic expression, etc.

So it's better to prevent these health issues before it arises.

**<u>SO, STOP SMOKING! LIVE A HEALTHY LIFE!
EVEN IF NOT FOR YOU,
FOR YOUR FAMILY!</u>**

www.ingramcontent.com/pod-product-compliance
Lightning Source LLC
Chambersburg PA
CBHW040249220526
45473CB00001B/423